EZ ECGs

Second Edition

Booklet

Written by
Cindy Tait
RN, MPH, CEN, CCRN

Center for Healthcare Education, Inc.
Riverside, California

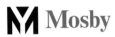

Mosby

A Harcourt Health Sciences Company

Publishing Director: Andrew Allen
Executive Editor: Claire Merrick
Developmental/Managing Editor: Kelly Trakalo
Project Manager: Gayle Morris

Printed in the United States of America

Mosby, Inc.
11830 Westline Industrial Drive
St. Louis, MO 63146

ISBN 0-323-01330-9

PREFACE

ECG interpretation was once a specialty skill used only by physicians and nurses working with critically ill cardiac patients. Increasingly over the past two decades the ability to accurately interpret cardiac dysrhythmias has become a requirement of healthcare providers working in a variety of clinical settings. Routine ECG monitoring is now a standard of care for patients with cardiac-related problems. Additionally, cardiac monitoring is beneficial for monitoring patients with acute or chronic diseases or traumatic injuries.

The most recent standards established by the American Heart Association emphasize early recognition and treatment of life-threatening dysrhythmias. Accurate ECG interpretation is the first step in identifying these dysrhythmias and ultimately reducing the morbidity and mortality of greater numbers of people. Combined with good assessment skills, the ECG can provide useful information to help you choose a treatment plan for optimal patient outcome.

The *EZ ECGs* videotape and booklet were designed to assist the beginning student with the fundamentals of basic ECG interpretation. The *EZ ECGs* program can be used as a resource and review for the healthcare provider already interpreting ECGs within his or her practice.

The emphasis of this program is twofold. The first objective is to provide you with the criteria to identify rhythms originating from the sinus node. The second is to present the most commonly encountered serious and/or lethal dysrhythmias—i.e., rhythms that often require immediate action to minimize or prevent an adverse patient response. Therefore, not all ECG rhythms will be presented in this program. You may want to supplement your ECG interpretation knowledge and skills by consulting other references.

Case studies with rhythm strips are presented to provide you with scenarios similar to those you may encounter in your practice. Emphasis should always be placed on treating the patient as a whole—and not just treating the monitor. ECG interpretation skills will complement your clinical assessment skills.

Keep in mind that ECG interpretation requires memorizing and understanding the specific criteria for each dysrhythmia. It is also a skill that requires frequent review and practice, as well as application in the clinical setting. Periodically review the criteria outlined in the booklet and test your skills using the scenarios in the videotape. The *EZ ECGs* program will help you build a solid foundation in the art and science of ECG interpretation.

The human heart is an amazing and wonderfully designed organ. This program will help you to better understand how it works and how to recognize and treat its diseases. I hope you will find this program enjoyable, easy to understand, and beneficial to your practice.

Cindy Tait
cindy@healthcareeducation.org

CONTENTS

SECTION FOUR

SECTION FIVE

CONTINUING EDUCATION CREDIT QUESTIONS . . 97

SECTION ONE

HOW TO USE THIS BOOKLET

The Cardiac Conduction System
Interpretation Tools
Important Terminology
Standard ECG Abbreviations

HOW TO USE THIS BOOKLET

The goal of the *EZ ECGs* program is to provide you with specific criteria and interpretation techniques to help you differentiate between normal, abnormal, and life-threatening ECG rhythms.

This booklet serves as a complement to the video program. It offers the practice of reading ECGs from printed strips whereas the video will teach you how to read dynamic, "on the fly" strips—a skill that is necessary for bedside patient monitoring. Before watching the video, review the cardiac anatomy, conduction system, waveform criteria, and interpretation tips found in Section One of this booklet. The video will then further reinforce the criteria that will help you to correctly identify sinus, atrial, junctional, and ventricular dysrhythmias.

The *EZ ECGs* booklet elaborates on information in the video. You may find it helpful to stop the video occasionally and review the related section in the booklet.

It is important to have a firm grasp of each concept and memorize the criteria before moving on to the next topic. Much of the frustration of learning to interpret ECGs can be eliminated by digesting the information in small segments.

A glossary of terms begins on page 20. Review each term before watching the video. If a word used in the video is new to you, jot it down so that you can look it up in the glossary. A working knowledge of ECG terminology will improve your ability to document your patient's dysrhythmias and help you report your findings to other members of the healthcare team.

Section Two presents the criteria for identifying rhythms that originate from the sinus node. It is important to be able to identify the normally conducted ECG rhythms. Once you are able to recognize the sinus rhythms, you will find it easier to identify many of the abnormal ECG rhythms that originate from other areas in the heart. By knowing the ECG rhythms originating from the sinus node, you will be able to better recognize when the heart's conduction system is healthy (e.g., a sinus bradycardia in an athlete) or when it is compensating for a disease state (e.g., sinus tachycardia in a patient in hypovolemic shock).

Section Three outlines the criteria for dysrhythmias that originate outside of the sinus node. These dysrhythmias are divided into sections based on their anatomic location in the heart and are placed into the categories of atrial, junctional, and ventricular. Many of the dysrhythmias are further categorized as either ectopic, escape, or blocked rhythms.

Section Four is to be used in conjunction with the scenarios presented on the videotape. Open the booklet to

this section as the scenarios are shown in the videotape so that you have a static copy of the rhythm and
patient information in front of you. You may want to
stop the tape to allow you to take your time. The exact
same strips are shown in the booklet and the video so
that you can evaluate the waveforms more closely and
measure the intervals. Also, by learning to interpret
dynamic rhythms from the videotape and static
rhythms from the booklet, you will become more ver-
satile in your ability to interpret ECGs in a variety of
patient care settings.

Section Five includes a comprehensive quiz to test your
ECG knowledge and interpretation skills. Complete and
mail in the posttest to receive 4 hours of approved continuing education credit for an additional fee.

Since you may not encounter all of the rhythms presented in this program on a regular basis, occasional
review will help you maintain and improve your ECG
skills. Keep this handy *EZ ECGs* booklet with you as a
quick reference guide to help you gain confidence and
competence in your ECG skills.

THE CARDIAC CONDUCTION SYSTEM

The metabolic processes of the human body depend on
the ability of the heart to pump oxygenated blood and
nutrients to the tissues. Movement of blood through
the cardiovascular system is accomplished when the
heart muscles respond to electrical stimulation by contracting. Blood enters the heart through the atrial
chambers. The right atrium receives blood from the
vena cava and pumps it into the right ventricle. The
right ventricle pumps blood into the pulmonary circulation. The left atrium receives the oxygenated blood
from the pulmonary system and pumps it into the left

ventricle and out through the aorta into the systemic circulation. This completes the circuit of providing blood and nutrients to the body's organs and tissues. (see Fig. 1-1).

Normal blood flow

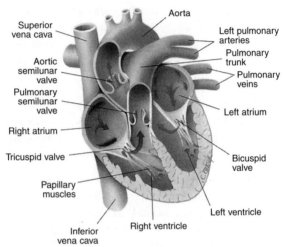

Fig. 1-1. Circulation through the heart. (From Sanders, MJ: Mosby's Paramedic Textbook, St. Louis, 1994, Mosby.)

The heart contains two specialized types of cells:

1. Working cells. The working cells of the heart are the muscular portions of the atria and ventricles. The heart muscle is called the *myocardium*. When properly stimulated by an electrical impulse, the working cells contract synchronously and pump blood to the lungs and tissues of the body. The status of the working cells can be evaluated by assessing the patient's hemodynamic status—i.e., pulse, blood pressure, skin perfusion, urine output, and level of consciousness.

2. Conduction cells. Electrical impulses are transmitted through the heart via specialized conduction cells. During a normal cardiac cycle electrical impulses begin in the sinoatrial (SA) node. The impulse is relayed to the atrioventricular (AV) node, where the impulse is delayed long enough to allow the blood to flow from the atria to the ventricles. The electrical impulse is then rapidly transmitted down the bundle branches and terminates in the Purkinje fibers implanted within the myocardium. The working cells respond to the stimulation by contracting. The speed of these impulses determine the heart rate. The heart rate is primarily influenced by the autonomic nervous system's response to the demands of the body for oxygenated blood. The status of the conduction system can be evaluated by interpreting the various components of the ECG tracing.

The cardiac conduction system consists of the sinoatrial (SA) node, the interatrial and internodal conduction tracts, the atrioventricular (AV) node, the bundle of His (also called the *AV junction*), the left and right bundle branches, and the Purkinje fibers, as seen in Fig. 1-2. Each node or region is capable of acting as the pacemaker of the heart. Should the SA node fail to act as the primary pacemaker, another site within the conduction system often takes over. This scenario is called an *escape pacemaker*. As a general rule, the further down the conduction system, the slower the rate of the escape rhythm and the wider the complex. The inherent rate for each site is shown in Fig. 1-3.

SA node	• 60 to 100 beats per min.
AV junction	• 40 to 60 beats per min.
Purkinje fibers	• 20 to 40 beats per min.

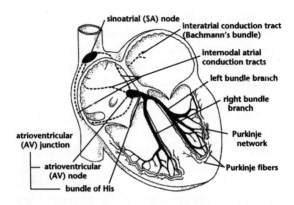

Fig. 1-2. Anatomy of the cardiac conduction system. (From Huzar RJ: Basic dysrhythmias: interpretation and management, 2e, St. Louis, 1994, Mosby.)

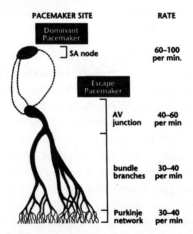

Fig. 1-3. Dominant and escape pacemakers. (From Huzar RJ: Basic dysrhythmias: interpretation and management, 2e, St. Louis, 1994, Mosby.)

Each ECG waveform represents electrical activity within a specific area of the heart. Knowing which waveform correlates with each area of the cardiac conduction system will help you to differentiate normal from abnormal conduction. A complete cardiac cycle has five identifiable waveforms. These electrical impulse patterns are labeled the P, Q, R, S, and T waves (Fig. 1-4).

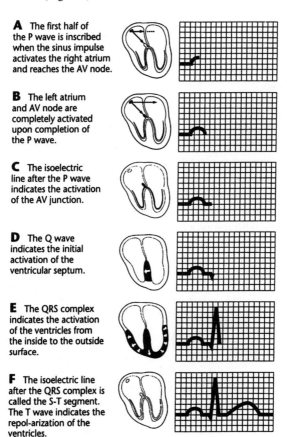

A The first half of the P wave is inscribed when the sinus impulse activates the right atrium and reaches the AV node.

B The left atrium and AV node are completely activated upon completion of the P wave.

C The isoelectric line after the P wave indicates the activation of the AV junction.

D The Q wave indicates the initial activation of the ventricular septum.

E The QRS complex indicates the activation of the ventricles from the inside to the outside surface.

F The isoelectric line after the QRS complex is called the S-T segment. The T wave indicates the repol-arization of the ventricles.

Fig. 1-4. Cardiac activation and ECG. (From Conover MS: Understanding electrocardiography: arrythmias and the 12-lead ECG, St. Louis, 1992, Mosby.)

In the commonly used perspective of lead II, normal
criteria for each waveform is defined as follows:

P wave represents depolarization of both atria. In lead
II, a normal P wave will be upright and rounded. The
P wave is identified as the first upright deflection from
the baseline (isoelectric line) at the beginning of the
cardiac cycle. Assuming your patient has a pulse, a
normal P wave indicates that the atrial chambers have
contracted and begun to empty blood into the ventricles.

QRS complex represents depolarization of the ventricles. The Q wave is the first negative deflection in the
cardiac cycle not preceded by an R wave. The R wave
is the first positive deflection in the QRS complex.
The S wave is the negative deflection that follows the
R wave. A normal QRS width is from 0.04 to 0.12
seconds in duration, or one to three small boxes wide.
The QRS complex is also referred to as the *systolic*, or
contraction, phase of the cardiac cycle. The QRS complex indicates the closing of the atrioventricular (AV)
valves, which creates the *lubb* sound during ausculta-

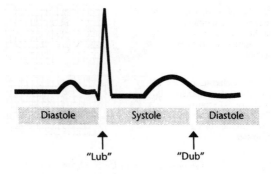

*Fig. 1-5. Systolic and diastolic phases of cardiac conduc-
tion.*

tion of the heart (see Fig. 1-5). It is important to note that you should feel a pulse with each QRS complex.

T wave represents the repolarization of the ventricles. The T wave is the first upward deviation after the brief isoelectric segment following the S wave. A normal T wave will be rounded and should not be notched or peaked. It is during the T wave that the ventricles are returning to an electrically ready state to receive the next impulse. The T wave is also referred to as the *diastolic*, or *resting*, phase of the cardiac cycle. The end of the T wave indicates closure of the pulmonic and aortic (semilunar) valves, which creates the *dubb* sound on auscultation.

After noting each waveform, it is important to identify and measure the intervals between the waveforms. Fig. 1-6 shows the beginning and endpoint of each interval.

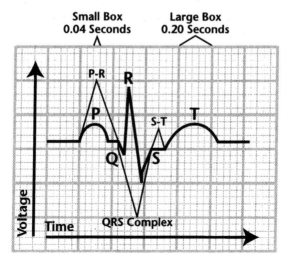

Fig. 1-6. Components of the ECG waveforms.

The first interval in the cardiac cycle is the P-R interval, which represents the transmission of an electrical impulse from the SA node to the atria to the AV junction. A normal P-R interval is 0.12 to 0.20 seconds, or three to five small boxes from beginning to end. A normal P-R interval indicates that conduction from the SA node to the AV node is free of obstruction or delays. Also, a normal P-R interval implies that the atrial chambers have had sufficient time to pump blood into the ventricles.

The second interval that you must evaluate is the S-T segment, which represents the start of the repolarization of the ventricles. The S-T segment begins with the completion of the S wave and ends with the beginning of the T wave. A normal S-T segment is flat and relatively close to the baseline (also called the *isoelectric line*). An S-T segment that is significantly above or below the baseline may indicate myocardial ischemia, an old or new myocardial infarction, cardiac disease, or effects of certain medications.

The R-to-R interval represents the time from one cardiac cycle to the next cycle. The R-to-R interval is measured from the peak of any given R wave to the peak of the next R wave. The heart rate directly affects the R-to-R interval. For example, the faster the heart rate, the shorter the R-to-R interval. A normal heart rate of 60 to 100 beats per minute will have three to five large boxes between R waves. Measure and compare at least three R-to-R intervals within the rhythm to determine whether the rhythm is regular or irregular (Figs. 1-7a and 1-7b).

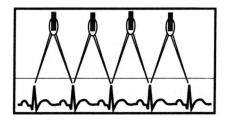

Fig. 1-7a. Regular R-R intervals.

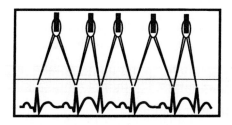

Fig. 1-7b. Irregular R-R intervals.

INTERPRETATION TOOLS

ECG paper is designed with a grid to provide a guide
for measuring the amplitude and length of the waveforms and intervals. Standard ECG paper is composed
of small boxes of 0.04 seconds each and large boxes
consisting of five small boxes that total 0.20 seconds
each. The large boxes are inscribed with a heavier line
(Fig. 1-8). Five consecutive large boxes equal 1 second. Most ECG paper is marked at the top with a vertical slash or an arrow indicating 1-second and/or 3-
second intervals. Each of these time intervals is helpful in determining the heart rate. The ECG recorder is
set at a standard speed of 25 mm per second. The tracing on the ECG graph paper is produced by a heated
stylus that literally burns the waveforms onto the
paper. The stylus moves up and down on the graph
paper in response to the electrical stimulus received.

ECG Leads

Electrical impulses traveling through the cardiac conduction system can be monitored by attaching elec-

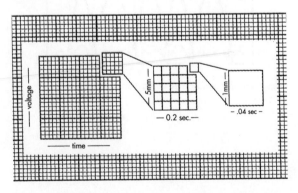

*Fig. 1-8. ECG paper (From Aehlert: ECGs Made Easy,
St. Louis, 1995, Mosby.)*

trodes to the surface of the skin. Electrical impulses traveling toward the *positive* electrode will result in an *upward* deflection on the ECG paper (Fig. 1-9). An impulse traveling toward the *negative* electrode will result in a *downward* deflection on the ECG paper. When there is no electrical activity in the heart, or if the electrical forces are equally positive and negative, the ECG tracing will show a flat line. This line is called the *isoelectric line*, or *baseline*. The best indicator of the true isoelectric line is the tracing between the T and the P waves. The isoelectric line is used as a reference point to determine whether other waveforms are depressed or elevated, a concept that is more commonly used in 12-lead ECG interpretation. The *ground* electrode is a safety feature that has a zero electrical potential. The *ground* lead helps to eliminate extraneous electrical interference from entering the monitor circuit.

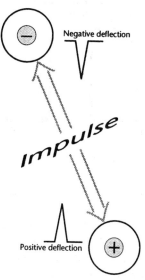

Fig. 1-9. Principles of electrical flow.

The most commonly used leads for field or routine bedside monitoring are leads I, II, III, MCL_1 and MCL_6. These leads can be established by arranging a positive, negative, and ground lead in the configuration shown in Fig. 1-10.

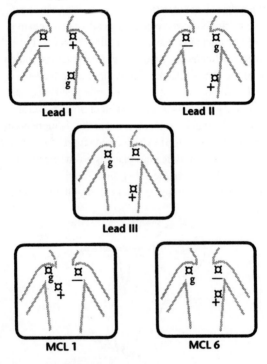

Lead I **Lead II**

Lead III

MCL 1 **MCL 6**

Fig. 1-10. Lead placement.

Each lead accentuates certain parts of the tracing. It is best to find a lead that will give you a clear tracing with prominent waveforms. Lead II and MCL_1 are the most commonly used continuous monitoring leads since they typically provide the most information about the waveforms and intervals. The *EZ ECGs* program displays all of the ECG rhythms in lead II.

Occasionally you may have difficulty getting a clear tracing on the ECG paper. Any marking on the ECG paper that is not directly related to cardiac conduction is called *artifact*. Many factors can contribute to artifact. Fig. 1-11 lists some troubleshooting tips for reducing outside interference. In some cases artifact may mimic a life-threatening dysrhythmia. Therefore, it is important to always eliminate the possibility of artifact and check your patient's status prior to treating any dysrhythmia.

Artifacts are distortions that obscure the cardiac impulse on the ECG tracing. Artifact may be caused by electrical, mechanical or patient interference. This often makes accurate interpretation difficult. Artifact may appear similar to a life-threatening dysrhythmia. Remember, the "patient is always right." Be sure to check the status of your patient before initiating any electrical or drug therapy. Listed below are a few tips for eliminating unwanted artifact:

Patient Preparation:	*Check for and correct:*
Explain procedure	Amplitude of gain
Preserve modesty	Lead selection
Dry skin	Dry electrode gel
Remove hair	Loose electrodes
Gently abrade and clean skin	Lead wire connection
Insure personal and patient safety	Damage to lead wires
	Improper electrode placement
	Patient movement
	T wave amplitude greater than R wave
	60-cycle interference

Fig. 1-11. ECG troubleshooting.

Rate Calculation

An important part of interpreting ECG rhythms is to
determine the heart rate. Heart rate is often a factor
used to determine whether a patient is stable or unsta-
ble. It is also an important criterion for choosing medications or electrical therapy. A heart that is beating
too slow may not be pumping enough blood to supply
the body's needs. When the heart is beating *too fast*
the ventricles and coronary arteries do not have sufficient time to adequately fill. This results in a
decreased cardiac output and myocardial ischemia.

A concept you should always remember is that each
QRS complex should generate a pulse. The only way
to determine whether each QRS complex is corresponding to actual movement of blood through the heart is
to take a pulse and simultaneously watch the ECG
monitor.

Most ECG monitoring machines are now equipped
with an electronic digital display of the heart rate. This
is helpful only during actual "live" monitoring of a
patient with a corresponding pulse. You may not
always be able to rely on the monitor and will have to
determine the heart rate using the ECG strip. There are
many methods and shortcuts for determining the heart
rate using the ECG graph paper and intervals of the
cardiac cycles.

A quick and simple method is to count the number of
R waves found in a 6-second strip and multiply by 10.
This will provide you with a "ballpark" estimate of the
rate per minute.

Keep in mind that in some dysrhythmias, the rates of
the atria and ventricles may differ. In other words, the

P waves may have a different rate than the QRS complexes. When this occurs, you will need to calculate
the rate of each. There are two calculation methods
that involve evaluating the R-to-R interval. The first is
the triplicate method, which is considered accurate
only if the overall rhythm is regular. To use this
method:

1. Select an R wave that lands on a dark vertical
   line on the ECG paper.
2. Count the large boxes" from left to right. Memorize the numbers 300, 150, 100, 75, 60, and 50
   consecutively.
3. You may need to estimate the rate if the second
   R wave lands in the middle of a large box. See
   example in Fig. 1-12 on page 18.

Five-Step Rhythm Analysis

At first glance some ECG rhythms may be intimidat-
ing. By approaching each rhythm strip using the five-
step rhythm analysis method, you will soon become
proficient at evaluating the criteria necessary to identify most rhythms. The five steps are:

1. Calculate the **QRS rate.**
2. Assess the regularity of the **rhythm.**
3. Determine the **QRS width.**
4. Evaluate the **atrial activity.**
5. Observe the **P-to-QRS relationship.**

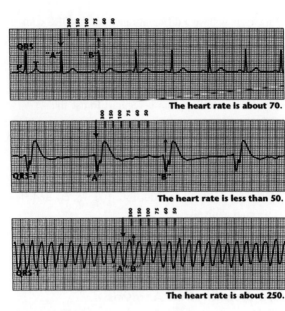

Fig. 1-12. Triplicate method. (From Huzar RJ: Basic dysrhythmias: interpretation and management, 2e, St. Louis, 1994, Mosby.)

1. Calculate the **rate of the QRS** complexes. If you are bedside with the patient, is it important to check the pulse and determine whether it correlates with the QRS rate. If there are more or less P waves than QRS complexes, then also calculate the rate of the P waves.

2. Observe the **rhythm** for at least 20 to 30 seconds and determine whether the rhythm is regular or irregular. Most authorities agree that the R-to-R intervals may vary as much as 0.04 seconds and the rhythm is still considered regular.

3. Measure the **width of the QRS** complex. A normal QRS complex is less than 0.12 seconds wide. A QRS complex wider than 0.12 seconds may be the result of a block or delay located in the bundle branches. A wide QRS complex may also indicate that the source of the rhythm is a ventricular impulse.

4. The P waves reflect the **atrial activity**. Compare the appearance and configuration of the P waves.

5. Observe the **relationship between the P waves and the QRS complexes**. There should be only one P wave for each QRS complex. Some dysrhythmias may have more P waves than QRS complexes. Next, measure the P-R interval. A normal P-R interval will be between 0.12 and 0.20 seconds long.

IMPORTANT TERMINOLOGY

Interpretation of ECGs includes communicating your findings with other healthcare personnel and documenting your interpretations. Knowledge of the terminology to most accurately describe ECG rhythms will facilitate these communications. Read through all the words in this guide and learn the terms that are new to you. You can also use this section as a glossary/dictionary reference. This list is only a partial compilation of ECG terms; you may need to refer to an ECG text or medical dictionary for words not included in this list.

Antiarrhythmic   Refers to medications that attempt to prevent or decrease the frequency of dysrhythmias and ectopic impulses.

Arteriosclerosis   Hardening and loss of elasticity of the arteries.

Asystole   Absence of electrical activity and contraction of the heart.

Atherosclerosis   A condition caused by an accumulation of debris along the intimal layer of the arteries.

Atrial kick   Filling of the ventricles with blood as a result of complete contraction and emptying of the atria.

AV block   Partial or complete obstruction of electrical impulses through the atrioventricular node. Categorized as first-, second-, or third-degree.

Bigeminy   Ectopic complexes occurring every other complex.

Bradycardia   A slow heart rate, typically less than 60 beats per minute.

Cadence   The pace and regularity of the cardiac rhythm.

Capture Depolarization of the heart; seen on ECG as a pacemaker spike followed by a wide QRS complex.

Cardiac cycle Includes the systolic and diastolic phases of the heart beat. A normal cycle includes the P, Q, R, S, and T waveforms.

Cardiac output The amount of blood pumped by the heart in one minute.

Compensatory pause A pause following a premature complex that allows the SA node to continue at its preset rhythm.

Conductivity The property of cardiac muscle cells to transmit electrical impulses.

Contractility The ability of the cardiac muscle cells to shorten when stimulated.

Controlled The ventricular rate is considered controlled if it is less than 100 beats per minute.

Couplet Two consecutive PVCs.

Depolarization The electrical process of discharging a resting cardiac cell.

Diastole The period of relaxation of the atria and ventricles. It is during this phase when the chambers of the heart and coronary arteries fill with blood.

Dysrhythmia Any ECG rhythm other than the normal sinus rhythm. May be benign or lethal.

Ectopic Refers to a beat or rhythm originating from a site other than the SA node. Ectopic beats are often premature.

Escape A complex or rhythm that is initiated when the underlying rhythm slows to less than the escape pacemaker's inherent rate.

Fibrillation Chaotic, uncoordinated electrical activity within the myocardium producing a quivering, ineffective muscular activity.

Flutter A regular pattern of electrical activity that displays a sawtooth appearance on the ECG.

Ground Electrode with a zero electrical potential that helps eliminate extraneous electrical interference.

Hemodynamic Refers to forces involved in perfusing the body with blood. Includes factors such as heart rate, force, preload, afterload, and vessel tone.

Hypertrophy Enlargement of a portion of the heart without an increase in chamber size.

Idioventricular Refers to a rhythm originating within the ventricles.

Infarction Necrotic tissue due to a sustained period of interrupted blood flow.

Inherent Refers to the rate at which a dominant or escape pacemaker normally initiates impulses.

Interval Measurable segment between ECG waveforms.

Ischemia Reduction in flow of oxygenated blood to a portion of cardiac tissue, which may be transient or irreversible.

Isoelectric Refers to a flat line on the ECG indicating no electrical activity or variations.

Joule A unit of electrical energy delivered through the chest wall for the purpose of synchronized cardioversion or defibrillation of the heart.

Junctional Term used to describe ectopic or escape rhythms originating within the AV junction.

Mobitz Name of the physician who identified two types of second-degree AV block.

Multifocal Term used to describe impulses that originate from multiple locations.

Myocardium Pertaining to the heart muscle, the working cells of the heart.

Necrosis Dead tissue resulting from an insufficient supply of oxygenated blood.

Parasympathetic Refers to the portion of the autonomic nervous system that produces slowing and depressing of cardiac function.

Paroxysmal   Term used to describe an abrupt onset of a dysrhythmia.

Perfusion   Flow of blood to tissues and/or organs.

Pulseless electrical activity   Electrical activity displayed on the ECG without evidence of mechanical response (no pulse).

Purkinje   Terminal portion of the cardiac conduction system embedded within the ventricles.

Quadrigeminy   Ectopic beat occurring every fourth complex.

Reentry   Circuit of ectopic beats caused by a single electrical impulse returning to a portion of tissue for a second or subsequent time.

Refractory   Inability to respond to an electrical stimulus because of incomplete repolarization.

Repolarization   Process by which a cell is restored to an electrically ready state.

Sinus   Pertaining to rhythms generated by the dominant pacemaker of the heart—the sinus node.

Supraventricular   Refers to the portion of the heart from the bundle branches to the SA node.

Sympathetic   Division of the autonomic nervous system responsible for stimulating cardiac activity.

Synchronize   Electrical shock timed to depolarize the entire myocardium. The shock will coincide with the R wave to prevent depolarization during the vulnerable T wave.

Systole   Contraction and subsequent movement of blood through the heart.

Tachycardia   Rapid heart rate, typically greater than 100 beats per minute.

Trigeminy   Ectopic complex arising every third beat.

Uncontrolled   Term used to describe a rhythm with a ventricular response greater than 100 beats per minute.

Unifocal   Arising from a single ectopic focus.

Vagal Refers to the tenth cranial (vagus) nerve, which influences heart rate and AV node conduction time by regulating parasympathetic tone.

Voltage The height and depth of a waveform measured in millimeters.

Watt/second See **joules.**

Wenckebach The name of the physician credited with discovering second-degree AV block type I.

Standard ECG Abbreviations

AIVR	accelerated idioventricular rhythm
AV	atrioventricular
BBB	bundle branch block
DC	direct current
ECG	electrocardiogram
EKG	electrocardiogram (German abbrev.)
f wave	fibrillatory wave
F wave	flutter wave
IVR	idioventricular rhythm
LBBB	left bundle branch block
MCL	modified chest lead
mV	millivolt
NSR	normal sinus rhythm (see **RSR**)
PAC	premature atrial complex
PAT	paroxysmal atrial tachycardia
PEA	pulseless electrical activity
PJC	premature junctional complex
PJT	paroxysmal junctional tachycardia
PVC	premature ventricular complex
RSR	regular sinus rhythm
RBBB	right bundle branch block
SA	sinoatrial
SVT	supraventricular tachycardia
VF	ventricular fibrillation
VT	ventricular tachycardia

WAP   wandering atrial pacemaker
1°AVBL first-degree AV block
2°AVBL second-degree AV block, types I or II
3°AVBL third-degree AV block

SECTION TWO

SINUS RHYTHMS

Normal Sinus Rhythm
Sinus Arrhythmia
Sinus Bradycardia
Sinus Tachycardia
Sinus Pause
Asystole
Pacemaker Rhythm

SINUS RHYTHMS

Standards have been established that define specific parameters for determining normal cardiac conduction. These standards include rates, waveform configurations, and intervals that are considered within "normal" limits for a healthy heart. The *normal sinus rhythm* is the basis, or reference point, by which all other rhythms are compared.

All sinus rhythms originate from the dominant pacemaker, the sinus node. Rhythms originating from outside the sinus node can be placed into one of three categories. These categories are defined by their location of origin and are labeled *atrial, junctional,* or *ventricular.*

Any rhythm that does not meet the criteria for normal sinus rhythm is called a *dysrhythmia.* The term *dys-*

rhythmia implies that there is a disturbance within the cardiac conduction system. Dysrhythmias have many implications, including acute or chronic cardiac disease or myocardial damage. The term *arrhythmia* is often used synonymously with the term *dysrhythmia*, although *arrhythmia* literally means "the absence of any rhythm." Section Three covers each dysrhythmia in detail.

This section will define the criteria for rhythms originating from the sinus node. Rhythm strip examples of the following sinus rhythms will be shown in lead II:

- Normal sinus rhythm
- Sinus arrhythmia
- Sinus bradycardia
- Sinus tachycardia
- Sinus pause
- Asystole
- Pacemaker rhythm

Throughout the booklet, each rhythm will be broken down into the categories used in the five-step rhythm analysis method. It is important to use this systematic approach with each rhythm you analyze.

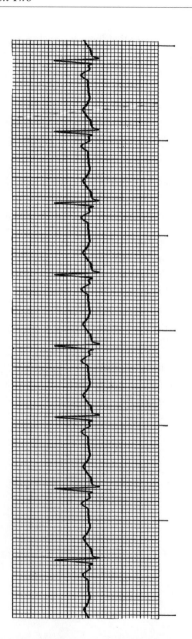

NORMAL SINUS RHYTHM

CRITERIA

Normal sinus rhythm, sometimes also called ***regular sinus rhythm,*** indicates that the pacing impulse is initiated within the sinus node and is transmitted normally down the conduction pathway.

QRS rate 60 to 100 beats per minute.

Rhythm Regular.

Atrial activity Normal and consistent P wave configuration.

QRS width 0.04 to 0.12 seconds.

P-to-QRS relationship 1:1 relationship with a P-R interval between 0.12 and 0.20 seconds.

Treatment When associated with a pulse, generally no treatment required.

The **"3 to 5 Rule"** states that a **Normal Sinus Rhythm** will have between:

3 to 5 small boxes in each P-R interval

3 to 5 large boxes in each R-R interval

SINUS ARRHYTHMIA

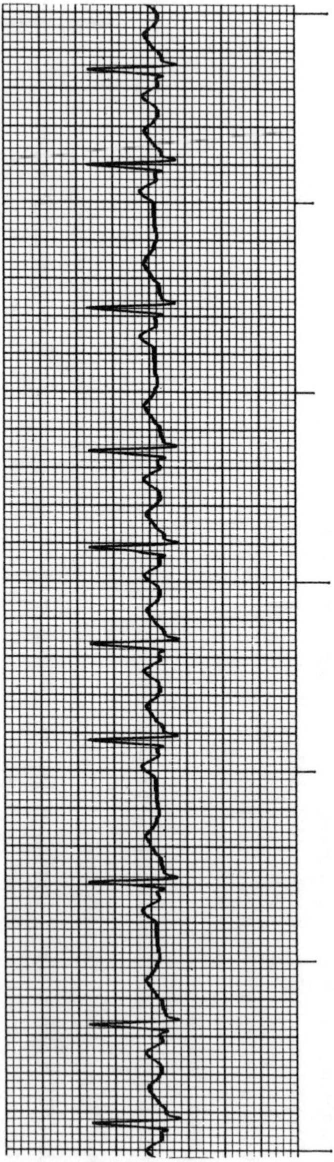

Sinus arrhythmia is a variation of normal sinus rhythm. It is common in children, healthy young adults, and the elderly. Sinus arrhythmia is usually caused by an inhibition of the vagus (parasympathetic) nerve during inspiration. A rhythmic pattern can be observed of an increase in heart rate during inspiration and a decrease in rate during expiration.

QRS rate   Usually 60 to 100 beats per minute.

Rhythm   Irregular.

Atrial activity   Normal and consistent P wave configuration.

QRS width   0.04 to 0.12 seconds.

P-to-QRS relationship   1:1 relationship with a P-R interval between 0.12 and 0.20 seconds.

Treatment   Usually no treatment is required unless the rate is slow and producing symptoms of inadequate cardiac output. In such cases atropine may be given to increase conduction throughout the AV node, or a pacemaker may be applied.

SINUS BRADYCARDIA

CRITERIA

Sinus bradycardia may be a normal rhythm in individuals with healthy hearts. Sinus bradycardia may also be a sign of acute or chronic heart disease, or it may be caused by an adverse reaction to medications that decrease the heart rate.

QRS rate   Less than 60 beats per minute.

Rhythm   Regular.

Atrial activity   Normal and consistent P wave configuration.

QRS width   0.04 to 0.12 seconds.

P-to-QRS relationship   1:1 relationship with a P-R interval between 0.12 and 0.20 seconds.

Treatment   Treatment is based on symptoms. If the patient is symptomatic of inadequate cardiac output, medications to increase heart rate such as atropine may be administered. In some situations a pacemaker may be required.

SINUS TACHYCARDIA

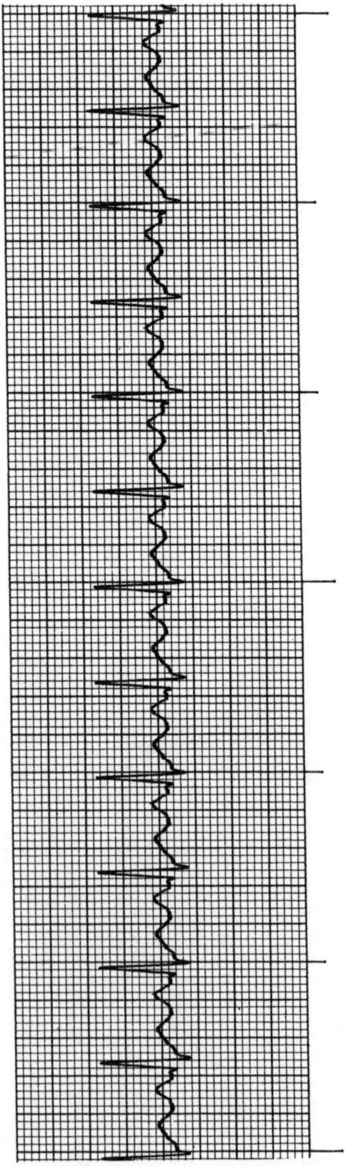

Sinus tachycardia is typically caused by an increase in the body's need of oxygenated blood such as during physical exertion, dehydration, fever, or shock. Sinus tachycardia may be a response to pain or fear. Occasionally, sinus tachycardia may be due to a myocardial infarction or congestive heart failure.

QRS rate   100 to 150 beats per minute.

Rhythm   Regular.

Atrial activity   Normal and consistent P wave configuration.

QRS width   0.04 to 0.12 seconds.

P-to-QRS relationship   1:1 relationship with a P-R interval between 0.12 and 0.20 seconds.

Treatment   Treatment should be focused on correcting the underlying cause. Oxygen therapy may be beneficial.

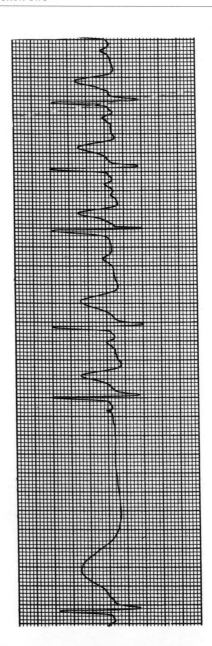

CRITERIA

Sinus pause may occur as a result of transient ischemia or permanent damage to the SA node. Sinus pause may also be caused by increased vagal (parasympathetic) tone, electrolyte imbalance, or an adverse effect of certain medications. The sinus node may fail to fire for one or more complexes.

QRS rate   Usually 60 to 100 beats per minute but may vary.

Rhythm   Irregular due to the pause (the underlying rhythm is often regular).

Atrial activity   Normal and consistent P wave configuration in the underlying rhythm. (Note: The rhythm after a pause may be an escape beat or rhythm.)

QRS width   0.04 to 0.12 seconds.

P-to-QRS relationship   1:1 relationship with a P-R interval of 0.12 and 0.20 seconds when sinus beats are present.

Treatment   Usually no treatment is indicated unless the patient shows signs of inadequate cardiac output. Further observation is advised.

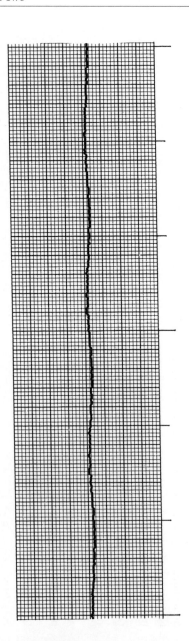

ASYSTOLE

CRITERIA

Asystole is the complete absence of sinus node or ventricular activity and is seen on the monitor as an uninterrupted horizontal line. Asystole is usually the terminal rhythm in cardiopulmonary arrest.

QRS rate None.

Rhythm None—only an isoelectric line.

Atrial activity None (occasionally nonconducted P-waves may be seen).

QRS width None.

P-to-QRS relationship None.

Treatment CPR; full resuscitation medications, including epinephrine and atropine.

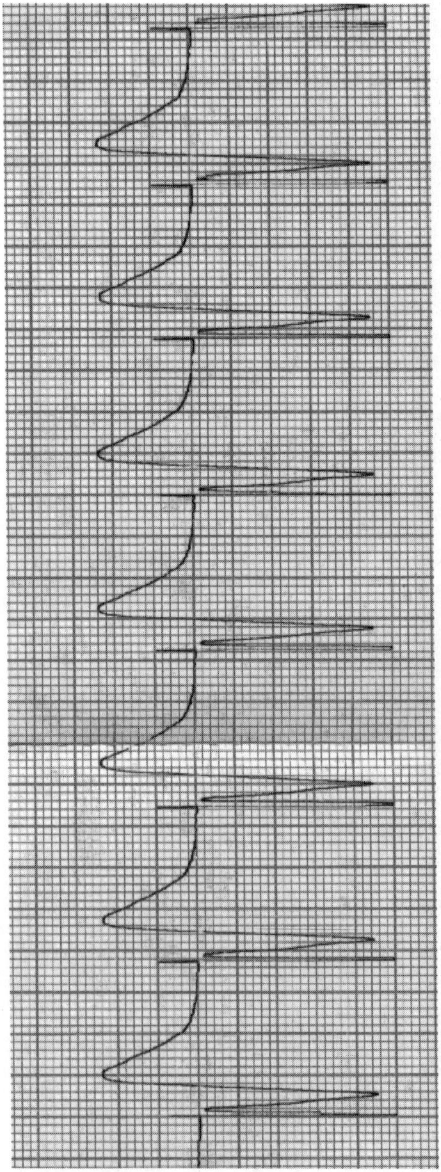

CRITERIA

Pacemaker rhythms will be seen on the ECG in patients for whom internal, transvenous cardiac pacemakers have been placed. There are many different types of pacemakers with many different settings; however, the hallmark of a pacemaker rhythm is a pacemaker "spike" before the QRS.

QRS rate   Rate is set by the physician, typically between 70 and 100 per minute.

Rhythm   May be regular or irregular, depending on involvement of the patient's own natural pacemaker.

Atrial activity   Absent when the pacemaker "captures." Atrial activity may be seen with the patient's own complexes.

QRS width   Captured complexes are wider than 0.14 seconds in duration.

P-to-QRS relationship   1:1—each pacemaker spike (if captured) will have a corresponding wide QRS complex.

Treatment   No treatment is required for properly functioning pacemakers.

SECTION THREE

DYSRHYTHMIAS

Etiologies of Dysrhythmias
Ectopic Beats and Rhythms
Atrioventricular Blocks
Escape Rhythms

DYSRHYTHMIAS

Now that you have an understanding of the rhythms
that originate from the sinus node, let's move on to
rhythms that are abnormally conducted. Disturbances
in cardiac conduction are called *dysrhythmias*. Dysrhythmias can occur even in healthy hearts. Often
minor dysrhythmias produce no symptoms and resolve
without any treatment. More serious dysrhythmias
indicate significant acute or chronic heart disease.
When serious dysrhythmias occur, medication is often
required to either speed up or slow down the ventricular rate, or to suppress an irritable area within the
myocardium. Occasionally, surgical intervention or
thrombolytic therapy is needed to prevent further damage and salvage any remaining viable heart tissue.
Dysrhythmias that are too fast or completely chaotic
may respond to the electrical therapy of cardiac pacing, synchronized cardioversion or defibrillation.

Once a dysrhythmia has been identified, you must
quickly and carefully assess your patient's vital signs
and general cardiovascular status. How well the

patient is tolerating the dysrhythmia and your hospital's protocols will determine how aggressively to treat the patient. It is important to know which interventions are best for his or her condition.

Etiologies of Dysrhythmias

ECG dysrhythmias may be benign or life-threatening. Dysrhythmias may arise from acute and reversible causes such as inadequate oxygenation. Dysrhythmias occurring during an acute event such as a myocardial infarction may be life-threatening. Other dysrhythmias are chronic and may be the result of extensive damage to the myocardial tissue and conduction system. Examples may include the following:

- coronary artery disease
- myocardial ischemia
- myocardial infarction
- digitalis toxicity
- fear, anxiety, or emotional stress
- electrolyte imbalance
- stimulants (caffeine, nicotine, etc.)
- left- or right-sided heart failure
- hypoxemia or acidosis
- drug overdose
- cardiomyopathies
- post–open heart surgery
- rheumatic fever
- electrical shock
- blunt or penetrating chest trauma
- right or left ventricular hypertrophy
- metabolic conditions (thyroid, anemia)
- chronic obstructive pulmonary disease
- valvular disease
- medications, including the following:
  - catecholamines

- beta blockers
- calcium channel blockers
- antiarrhythmics

Dysrhythmias can be evaluated from three viewpoints.

1. Ventricular response

Begin your ECG assessment by evaluating the ventricular response. The contraction of the ventricles determines most of the cardiac output and perfusion of blood to the lungs, organs, and body tissues. The ventricular rate can be determined by palpating a pulse that coincides with each QRS complex. The ventricular rate can be determined by counting the pulse rate. All of the new ECG monitors have a heart rate display and ability to print the heart rate on the ECG graph paper with other pertinent patient information. However, always make sure that your patient has a corresponding pulse, and report any disparities. Abnormal ventricular conduction can be viewed as being:

- Too fast
- Too slow
- Too irritable
- Lethal or absent

2. Origin of impulse

Dysrhythmias are placed into categories based on the anatomic location of the impulse formation. The prefix of the dysrhythmia will identify the origin as either:

- Atrial
- Junctional
- Ventricular

3. Electrophysiology of the impulse

The last component of your dysrhythmia evaluation is to look at the electrophysiology, or character, of the conduction disturbance. The *EZ ECGs* booklet places the dysrhythmias into groups based on similar distinguishing traits. The dysrhythmias will be categorized as:

- Ectopic beats
- Ectopic rhythms
- Atrioventricular blocks
- Escape rhythms

By applying the five-step rhythm analysis to the following rhythms, you will learn how to recognize many common dysrhythmias encountered in the clinical setting.

Ectopic Beats and Rhythms

An abnormal impulse formation may initiate an ectopic rhythm. The three predominant mechanisms that generate ectopic rhythms are:

- Reentry
- Enhanced automaticity
- Triggered activity

Reentry occurs when an electrical impulse is blocked or delayed in a portion of the conduction system. The interruption of impulses allow some of the unaffected cells time to repolarize. Once repolarized, the cells can be depolarized a subsequent time. This may result in a single (ectopic) beat or repetitive abnormal impulses (ectopic rhythm), which are often tachycardic. Reentry is commonly caused by ischemic heart disease, myocardial infarction, or electrolyte imbalances (Fig. 3-1).

Enhanced automaticity occurs when impulses from the pacemaker cells are altered. This causes either an enhancement of impulses from normal pacemaker cells or conflicting impulses arising from the same pacemaker site. The alteration and interference of

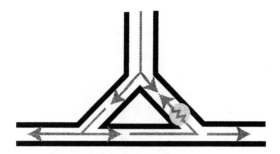

Fig. 3-1. Reentry.

impulses causes ectopic beats and rhythms. Enhanced automaticity can be caused by hypoxia, digitalis toxicity, electrolyte imbalances, ischemic heart disease, myocardial infarction, cardiomyopathies, or actions of cardiac medications.

Triggered activity occurs when pacemaker and/or nonpacemaker cells depolarize multiple times following a single electrical stimulation. Triggered activity is the result of "after depolarizations" that occur immediately after a cardiac cycle or just before the next cycle. This type of abnormal conduction can result in ectopic beats, runs of beats, or paroxysmal tachycardias. The causes of triggered activity are similar to enhanced automaticity.

Understanding the electrophysiology of a dysrhythmia is not as important as being able to correctly identify each dysrhythmia and respond with the appropriate interventions. Remember, *most of the lethal and life-threatening dysrhythmias are the easiest to identify.*

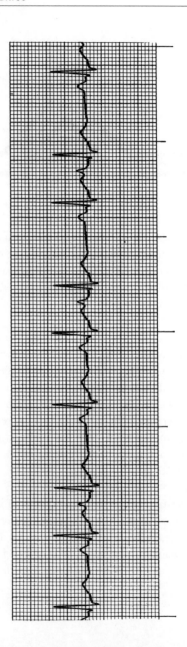

CRITERIA

Premature atrial complexes, abbreviated *PACs*, are isolated early beats that indicate an irritable focus within the atria. PACs may appear in healthy hearts or may indicate disease or damage within the atrial tissue. Often PACs are caused by stimulants such as emotional stress, caffeine, or nicotine.

QRS rate May occur at any heart rate.

Rhythm Irregular when PACs occur.

Atrial activity P waves may or may not be seen preceding the ectopic complex.

QRS width The QRS width is not usually affected by a PAC and will appear similar to the QRS complexes in the underlying rhythm.

P-to-QRS relationship 1:1 relationship for all complexes with observable P waves.

Treatment Often no treatment is required. Remove suspect stimulants. Evaluate for underlying heart disease and treat accordingly.

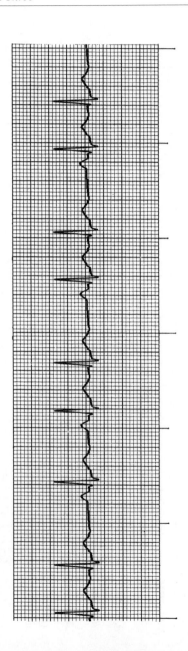

CRITERIA

Premature junctional complexes, abbreviated *PJCs*, are isolated early beats that indicate an irritable focus within the AV junction. PJCs may occur in healthy hearts without any obvious cause, but may be caused by disease involving the tissues of the AV junction. Certain medications may cause PJCs, most commonly digitalis.

QRS rate May occur at any heart rate.

Rhythm Irregular when PJCs occur.

Atrial activity P waves may appear before or after the QRS of the ectopic complex, or may be hidden within the QRS.

QRS width The QRS width is not usually affected by a PJC and will appear similar to the QRS complexes in the underlying rhythm.

P-to-QRS relationship 1:1 relationship for all complexes with observable P waves.

Treatment Often no treatment is required. Check for digitalis toxicity or other medications in nontherapeutic doses.

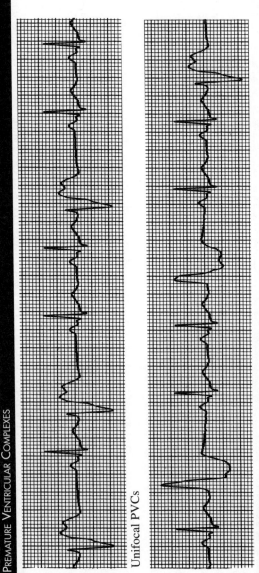

PREMATURE VENTRICULAR COMPLEXES

Unifocal PVCs

Multifocal PVCs

CRITERIA

Premature ventricular complexes, or *PVCs*, are early beats that indicate one or more irritable foci within the ventricles. PVCs that are similar in appearance indicate a single area or irritability and are called *unifocal PVCs*. PVCs that are different in appearance indicate more than one area of irritability and are called *multifocal PVCs*. PVCs may occur in healthy individuals and should not cause concern. PVCs often indicate ischemic heart disease, hypoxia, electrolyte imbalances, myocardial infarction, or an adverse response to certain medications.

QRS rate PVCs may occur at any heart rate.

Rhythm Irregular when PVCs occur.

Atrial activity P waves may or may not be seen preceding the ectopic complex.

QRS width The hallmark of PVCs is a QRS complex that is greater than 0.12 seconds.

P-to-QRS relationship There is no observable relationship between the P waves and the QRS complexes of PVCs.

Treatment Treatment of PVCs is based on the frequency and focus of the PVCs, as well as the presences of any associated symptoms. Treatment often includes antiarrhythmic drugs such as lidocaine and oxygen administration.

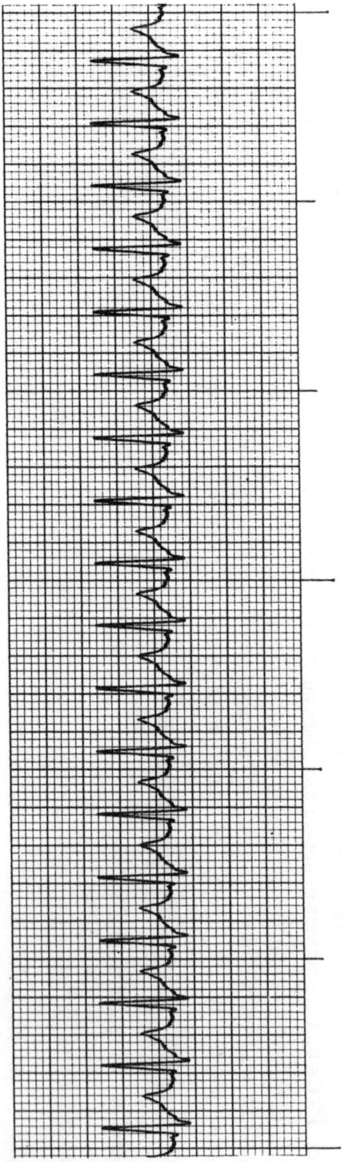

CRITERIA

Atrial tachycardia originates from an irritable focus within the atria. Atrial tachycardia frequently has an abrupt onset. This is called *paroxysmal atrial tachycardia (PAT)*. Atrial tachycardia is considered a supraventricular tachycardia (SVT or PSVT when paroxysmal). Atrial tachycardia is usually caused by ischemic heart disease, a myocardial infarction, or digitalis toxicity. Patients with atrial tachycardia often complain of feelings of palpitations or a fluttering sensation in their chest.

QRS rate 160 to 250.

Rhythm Regular.

Atrial activity P waves may or may not be visible.

QRS width 0.04 to 0.12 seconds.

P-to-QRS relationship Any visible P waves will usually have a 1:1 relationship with the QRS complexes.

Treatment Treatment may include vagal maneuvers, medications such as adenosine or verapamil, and/or synchronized cardioversion.

ATRIAL FLUTTER

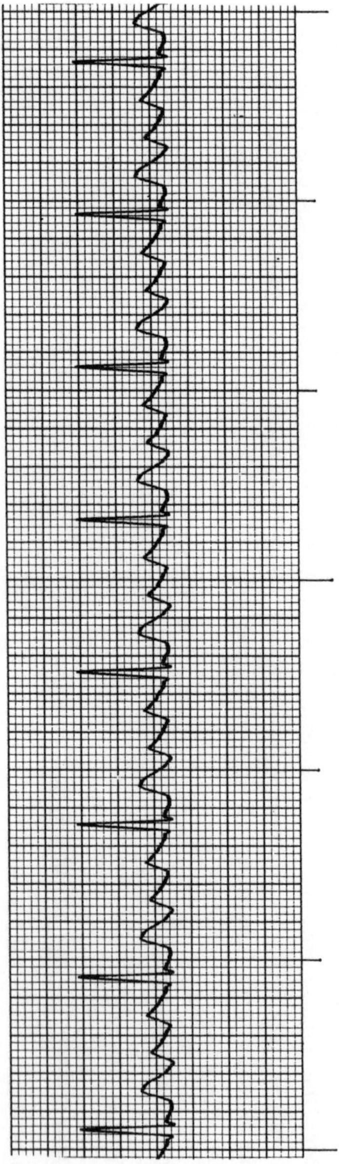

CRITERIA

Atrial flutter is most often caused by a reentry circuit within the atria. The identifying feature of this rhythm is the "picket fence" or "sawtooth" pattern F waves between the QRS complexes. The fluttering within the atria does not allow for complete emptying of the atrial chambers into the ventricles. This results in a reduction of about 25% of the cardiac output. Atrial flutter is seen in patients with rheumatic heart disease, valvular problems, and ischemic disease.

QRS rate May vary from slow to tachycardic. A rate below 100 per minute is labeled "controlled"; above 100 per minute is "uncontrolled."

Rhythm The atrial F waves will be regular. QRS rhythm may be regular or irregular.

Atrial activity Characteristic F waves with a rate of 250 to 350 per minute.

QRS width Usually normal at 0.04 to 0.12 seconds. F waves may coincide with some of the QRS complexes, causing some complexes to appear distorted.

P-to-QRS relationship F waves replace normal P waves and may have a 2:1, 3:1, or 4:1 relationship.

Treatment Treatment is based on the QRS rate and may include digitalis or cardioversion.

ATRIAL FIBRILLATION

CRITERIA

Atrial fibrillation is caused by enhanced automaticity or a reentry mechanism. The chaotic unorganized electrical activity within the atria cause the chambers to quiver ineffectively. This can reduce the cardiac output by as much as 25%. Atrial fibrillation is common in the elderly and individuals with coronary artery disease. It is frequently associated with congestive heart failure.

QRS rate The QRS rate may be "controlled" at less than 100 per minute, or "uncontrolled" at greater than 100 beats per minute.

Rhythm The QRS rhythm is typically irregular.

Atrial activity No discernible P waves. Atrial activity shows chaotic wavy "f waves."

QRS width 0.04 to 0.12 seconds.

P-to-QRS relationship None.

Treatment Treatment is based on the rate of the ventricular response and may include drugs such as digitalis, beta blockers, or synchronized cardioversion.

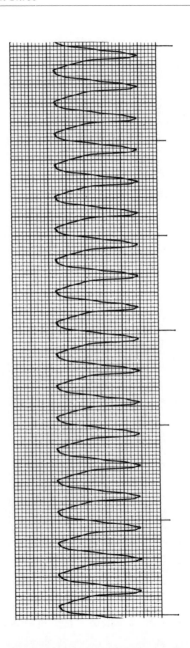

VENTRICULAR TACHYCARDIA

CRITERIA

Ventricular tachycardia (V-tach) is caused by an irritable focus within the Purkinje fibers or ventricular myocardium. Three or more PVCs in a row is considered ventricular tachycardia. V-tach may be attributed to hypoxia, electrolyte imbalances, or significant heart disease. V-tach is an ominous, life-threatening dysrhythmia that requires rapid intervention. Without treatment V-tach may quickly decline into V-fib.

QRS rate 100 to 250 per minute.

Rhythm Usually regular.

Atrial activity P waves may or may not be present.

QRS width Greater than 0.12 seconds.

P-to-QRS relationship None.

Treatment Treatment for V-tach is based on whether or not a pulse is present. If a pulse is present, treatment is based upon the patient's hemodynamic status. Antiarrhythmic medications such as lidocaine, procainamide, or bretylium may be administered. Other treatments may include synchronized cardioversion, defibrillation, and CPR.

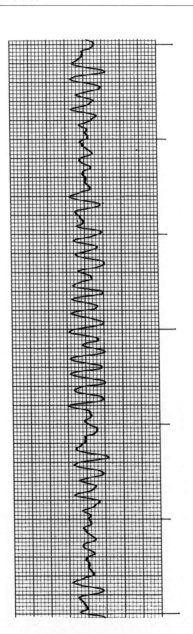

VENTRICULAR FIBRILLATION

CRITERIA

Ventricular fibrillation (V-fib) occurs when the cells of the ventricular myocardium depolarize in a chaotic and uncoordinated manner. No pulse can be felt during ventricular fibrillation because the heart is incapable of pumping blood. Causes of V-fib include acute myocardial infarction, electrolyte imbalances, hypoxia, and adverse reactions to medications.

QRS rate   None.

Rhythm   Chaotic.

Atrial activity   None.

QRS width   No discernable complexes can be observed. Fibrillatory waves may be coarse (large) or fine (small).

P-to-QRS relationship   None.

Treatment   Rapid defibrillation is the treatment of choice. CPR should be initiated until a defibrillator is available. Medications may include epinephrine, antiarrhythmics, and magnesium sulfate. Note: loose leads, patient movement, or artifact may mimic V-fib; therefore, it is important to always check the patient's hemodynamic status, lead attachment, and the monitor prior to implementing treatment.

Atrioventricular Blocks

Atrioventricular (AV) blocks occur when a portion of the cardiac conduction system is damaged. Ischemic, injured, or necrotic tissue can cause delayed or blocked conduction of electrical impulses. AV blocks typically produce slow ventricular rates. Treatment is often focused on increasing the heart rate until the cause can be corrected or a pacemaker applied. The key to identifying AV blocks is the P-to-QRS relationship. By determining the rate of the P waves, the ratio of P waves to QRS complexes and the P-R interval, you will be able to identify the block. AV blocks are placed into three categories based on the location and severity of the block (Fig. 3-2).

First-degree block is actually not a block but a delay in conduction through the AV node.

Second-degree blocks type I and II are more serious AV blocks that are located further down the cardiac conduction system. Second-degree blocks result in missed QRS complexes. This will be seen as either dropped QRS complexes or a P-to-QRS ratio of greater than 1:1.

Third-degree block, sometimes called *complete heart block*, indicates that the electrical impulses are completely blocked between the atria and the ventricles. Third-degree block indicates that the ventricles are responding to impulses generated within the lower portion of the AV junction or from the Purkinje fibers in the ventricles.

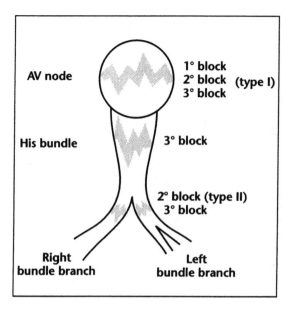

Fig. 3-2. Locations of AV blocks.

Another easy way to learn the three classifications of AV blocks is to remember:

In **First-Degree AV Block**,
"*All* of the beats go through"

In **Second-Degree AV Block**,
"Only *some* of the beats go through"

and

In **Third-Degree AV Block**,
"*None* of the beats go through"

FIRST-DEGREE AV BLOCK

CRITERIA

First-degree AV block is caused by a delay in conduction through the AV node. First-degree AV block may appear in healthy individuals without reason for concern. Other causes of first-degree block include digitalis toxicity, electrolyte imbalances, and myocardial ischemia or infarction. Certain medications may cause first-degree AV block by slowing conduction through the AV node.

QRS rate 60 to 100 per minute, occasionally bradycardic and less than 60 per minute.

Rhythm Regular.

Atrial activity Normal and consistent P wave configuration.

QRS width 0.04 to 0.12 seconds.

P-to-QRS relationship 1:1 relationship with a P-R interval greater than .20 seconds.

Treatment Usually no treatment is required unless the ventricular rate is less than 60 per minute resulting in an inadequate cardiac output.

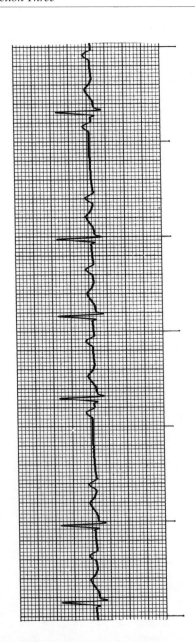

SECOND-DEGREE AV BLOCK TYPE I (WENCKEBACH/MOBITZ TYPE I)

CRITERIA

Second-degree AV block type I, also called ***Wenckebach*** or ***Mobitz type I,*** is caused by injury or damage within or just below the AV node. Second-degree type I is most commonly due to an inferior-wall myocardial infarction. Other causes includes digitalis toxicity, electrolyte imbalances, ischemic heart disease, or post–open heart surgery.

QRS rate   May occur at any rate.

Rhythm   Irregular. Note: the hallmark of this rhythm is groups of beats ending with a dropped beat.

Atrial activity   Normal and consistent P wave configuration.

QRS width   The QRS width is not affected by the block and will be 0.04 to 0.12 seconds.

P-to-QRS relationship   Beginning with each group of beats, the P-R interval will progressively lengthen until a QRS complex is dropped. This can be observed by a P wave without a subsequent QRS complex at the end of each group of beats.

Treatment   Usually no treatment is needed if the heart rate is adequate. Treat any underlying cause. If the block is related to an MI, it will often resolve within 72 to 96 hours.

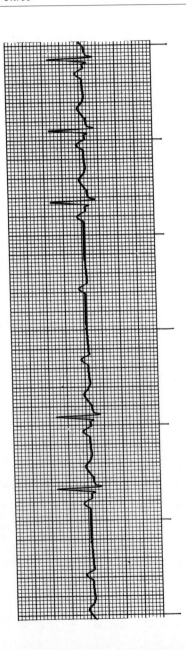

SECOND-DEGREE AV BLOCK TYPE II (MOBITZ TYPE II)

Second-degree AV block type II, also called ***Mobitz type II,*** is the more serious of the second-degree blocks. This block indicates damage within or below the AV junction with intermittent conduction through the bundle branches. Second-degree type II is usually the result of advanced heart disease, although it may be caused by digitalis toxicity. Second-degree type II rarely resolves without treatment.

QRS rate May occur at any rate. Most commonly produces slow ventricular rates.

Rhythm May be regular or irregular.

Atrial activity Normal and consistent appearing P waves.

QRS width May be normal at 0.04 to 0.12 seconds. If the block is located within the bundle branches, the QRS complex may be greater than 0.12 seconds.

P-to-QRS relationship P waves can be seen that do not conduct QRS complexes. This may occur at regular intervals (i.e., 2:1, 3:1, 4:1, etc.). P-R intervals will be constant with all conducted QRS complexes.

Treatment Treatment is based on the ventricular rate and cardiac output. This rhythm may not respond well to drugs and often requires a pacemaker.

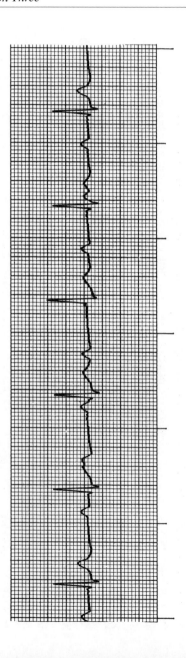

THIRD-DEGREE AV BLOCK (COMPLETE HEART BLOCK)

CRITERIA

Third-degree AV block, also called ***complete heart block***, is the result of a complete blockage of electrical impulses through the AV node and junction. In order for the heart to continue pumping, electrical impulses must be initiated by a junctional or ventricular escape pacemaker. Third-degree block with a ventricular escape rhythm is a potentially lethal rhythm that requires immediate action.

QRS rate The QRS rate is usually less than 60 per minute.

Rhythm Since the atria and ventricles are firing independently, the P waves and QRS complexes will have different rates (the P waves typically will have the faster rate).

Atrial activity Normal and consistent P wave configuration.

QRS width The QRS width will depend on the escape pacemaker and may be normal or wide (>0.12 seconds).

P-to-QRS relationship There is no relationship between the P waves and QRS complexes.

Treatment Treatment is based on the ventricular response rate and cardiac output. This block may not respond to medication and often requires a pacemaker. Close observation is advised.

Escape Rhythms

Escape rhythms occur when the normal pacemaker, the sinus node, fails to fire. An escape rhythm may also occur when the AV junction fails to fire at a rate faster than the inherent rate of the ventricles. An escape beat or rhythm may arise after a sinus pause. Third-degree (complete) AV blocks typically have either a junctional or ventricular escape rhythm.

The location of the escape rhythm is determined by the ventricular rate and the width of the QRS complexes. Obviously, the slower the rate, the greater the potential for decreased cardiac output. Also, the "atrial kick," the contribution of the blood actively pumped from the atria, is absent when escape rhythms or beats occur. The result is 20% to 30% less cardiac output.

Here are some rules to help you to differentiate the escape rhythms:

Junctional Escape
QRS rate—40 to 60 per minute
QRS width—narrow

Ventricular Escape
QRS rate—40 or less per minute
QRS width—wide

In **junctional escape** rhythms, the P waves may appear before or after the QRS complexes or may be hidden within the QRS complexes. The location of the block and speed of the impulses will determine the configuration of the P waves (Fig. 3-3).

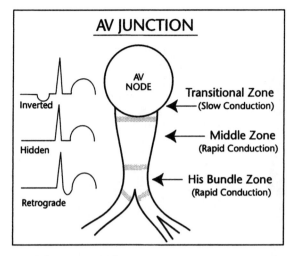

Fig. 3-3. P wave configurations.

Ventricular escape rhythms have wide and bizarre-shaped QRS complexes. Since these complexes originate from the ventricles, they appear similar to PVCs. However, a ventricular escape rhythm is not multiple PVCs! Ventricular escape occurs when impulses from all other higher pacemakers are blocked. Ventricular escape then becomes the only mechanism from which the heart can generate pacing impulses. Treatment for ventricular escape rhythm is focused on increasing the heart rate, whereas treatment for PVCs is directed toward reducing the irritable focus with antiarrhythmic medications.

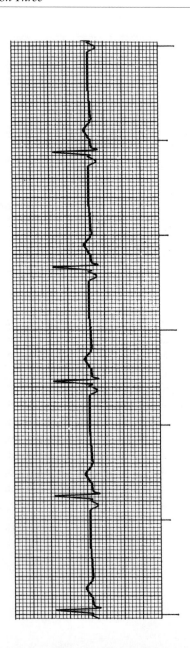

Junctional escape rhythm occurs when the SA node fails to fire when impulses are blocked at the level of the AV node. The AV junction will usually take over as the pacemaker within 1 to 1.5 seconds of not receiving an impulse from the SA node. Junctional escape rhythms may be caused by ischemia or injury involving the SA node, sick sinus syndrome, or digitalis toxicity.

QRS rate 40 to 60 per minute.

Rhythm Regular.

Atrial activity Inverted or absent P waves.

QRS width 0.04 to 0.12 seconds.

P-to-QRS relationship 1:1 relationship if P waves are present. P-R interval will be less than 0.12 seconds. P waves may be hidden within the QRS or appear after the QRS complexes. See Fig. 3-3.

Treatment If a slow ventricular rate is causing inadequate cardiac output, treatment will be directed toward increasing the rate with medication such as atropine or the application of a pacemaker. Close observation is advised.

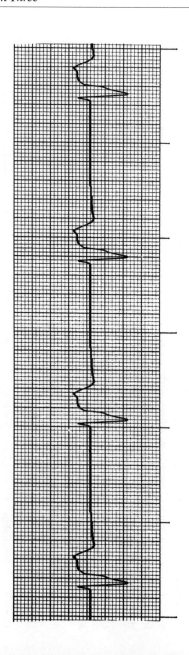

VENTRICULAR ESCAPE RHYTHM

Ventricular Escape Rhythm, also called ***idioventricular*** or ***agonal rhythm,*** is a safety mechanism by which the Purkinje fibers or ventricular myocardium initiate pacing impulses. This occurs when all of the impulses from the SA node or AV junction are absent or blocked. Ventricular escape is an ominous rhythm that may degenerate into asystole without rapid intervention.

QRS rate Less than 40 per minute.

Rhythm Regular.

Atrial activity Usually none. Occasional, infrequent P waves may appear throughout the rhythm.

QRS width Greater than 0.12 seconds.

P-to-QRS relationship None.

Treatment Treatment is directed toward increasing the ventricular rate. This rhythm may or may not respond to atropine or other medications and will usually require the application of a pacemaker.

SCENARIOS

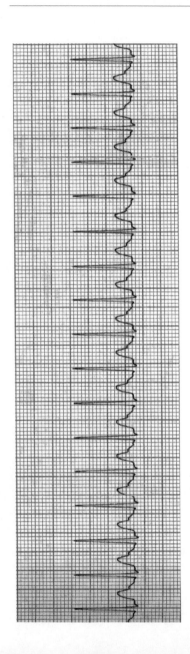

Scenario 1
27-year-old female

Pulse: 180 per minute, regular
Respirations: 26 per minute
Blood pressure: 102/62

History: Stress, caffeine, nicotine
Medication: Oral birth control

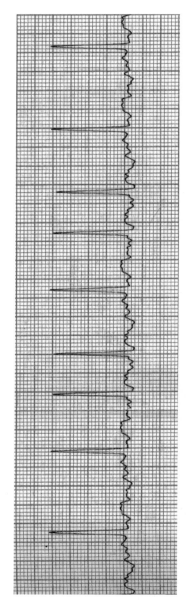

Scenario 2
72-year-old male

Pulse: 90 per minute, irregular
Respirations: 20 per minute
Blood pressure: 160/84

History: Hernia, MI three years ago
Medication: Lasix, digoxin

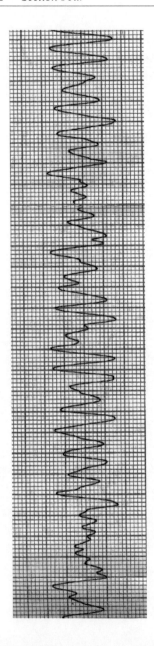

Scenario 3
Elderly male

Pulse: No pulse
Respirations: Assisted with bag-valve-mask
Blood pressure: None

History: Unknown
Medication: Unknown

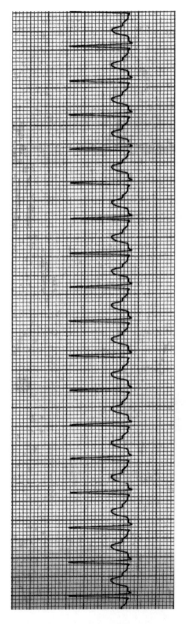

Scenario 4
25-year-old female

Pulse: 198 per minute, strong, regular
Respirations: 24 per minute
Blood pressure: 102/56

History: 22 weeks pregnant
Medication: Prenatal vitamins

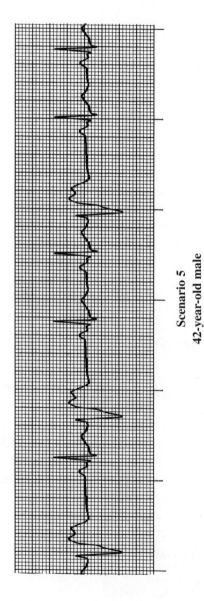

Scenario 5
42-year-old male

History: Asthma, acute substernal chest pain
Medication: Ventolin inhaler

Pulse: 98 per minute, regular
Respirations: 24 per minute with expiratory wheezes
Blood pressure: 136/80

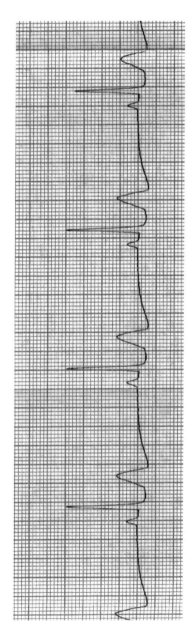

Scenario 6
32-year-old female

Pulse: 40 per minute, regular
Respirations: 6 per minute and assisted
Blood pressure: 100/40

History: Suspected barbiturate overdose
Medication: Unknown

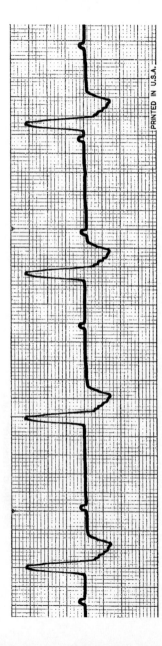

Scenario 7
92-year-old male

Pulse: 50 per minute, regular
Respirations: 18 per minute
Blood pressure: 118/82

History: Stroke, two previous MIs, semiconscious
Medication: Inderal, Zantac

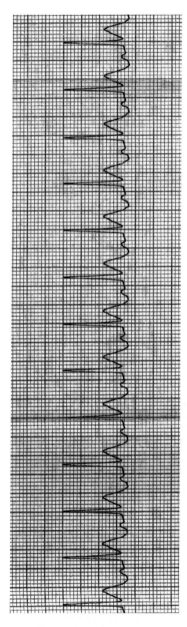

Scenario 8
23-year-old male

Pulse: 150 per minute, regular
Respirations: 26 per minute
Blood pressure: 112/78

History: Bleeding laceration
Medication: None

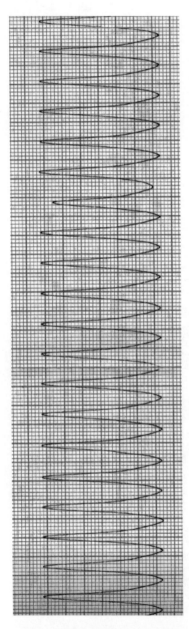

Scenario 9
59-year-old male

Pulse: None
Respirations: None
Blood pressure: Unknown

History: Being transferred for open heart surgery
Medication: Multiple cardiac medications, vasopressors

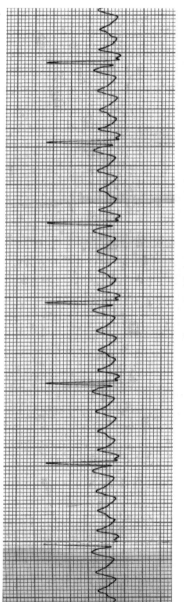

Scenario 10
80-year-old male

Pulse: 80 per minute, slightly irregular
Respirations: 18 per minute and clear
Blood pressure: 173/93

History: Possible stroke
Medication: Coumadin

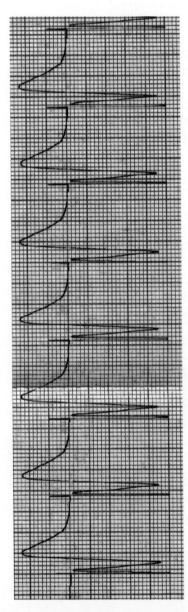

Scenario 11
71-year-old female

Pulse: 72 per minute, regular
Respirations: 16 per minute
Blood pressure: 140/78

History: Two previous MIs, diabetes
Medication: Oral diabetic and cardiac medications

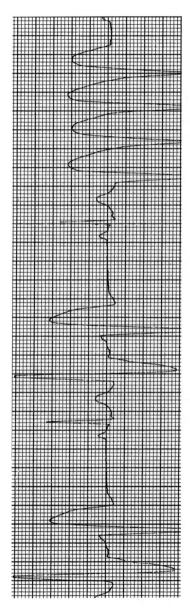

Scenario 12
47-year-old male

Pulse: 62 per minute, irregular
Respirations: 22 per minute and labored
Blood pressure: 98/52

History: None
Medication: None

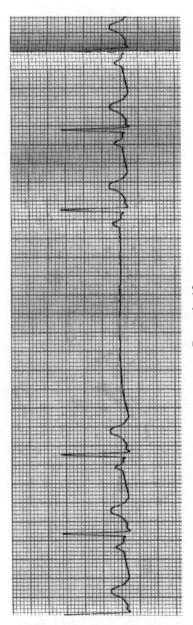

Scenario 13
Male

Pulse: 38 per minute, very irregular

Respirations: 32 per minute and shallow

Blood pressure: 82/40

History: None

Medication: None

SECTION FIVE

PRACTICE SELF-TEST QUESTIONS

1. The branch of the autonomic nervous system that slows the heart rate is the:
   a. sympathetic.
   b. parasympathetic.
   c. inotropic.
   d. chronotropic.

2. The P wave represents the firing of the:
   a. SA node.
   b. AV node.
   c. Purkinje fibers.
   d. ventricular myocardium.

3. The QRS complex represents:
   a. atrial depolarization.
   b. normal delay in the AV node.
   c. ventricular depolarization.
   d. ventricular repolarization.

4. The T wave represents:
   a. atrial repolarization.
   b. atrial depolarization.
   c. ventricular repolarization.
   d. ventricular depolarization.

5. Which heart rate is considered bradycardia?
   a. Less than 150 per minute
   b. Less than 100 per minute
   c. Less than 80 per minute
   d. Less than 60 per minute

6. Which heart rate is typical of atrial tachycardia?
   a. 100 to 150 per minute
   b. 160 to 250 per minute
   c. 200 to 350 per minute
   d. Greater than 350 per minute

7. What is the normal P-R interval?
   a. 0.12 to 0.20 seconds
   b. 0.04 to 0.12 seconds
   c. 0.04 to 0.20 seconds
   d. Greater than 0.20 seconds

8. What is the normal QRS width?
   a. 0.12 to 0.20 seconds
   b. 0.04 to 0.12 seconds
   c. 0.04 to 0.20 seconds
   d. Greater than 0.20 seconds

9. Indicators of the adequacy of cardiac output include:
   a. blood pressure.
   b. mental status.
   c. urine output.
   d. pulse.
   e. all of the above.

10. One small box on the ECG graph paper equals:
    a. 0.20 seconds.
    b. 0.04 seconds.
    c. 1 second.
    d. 3 seconds.

11. One large box on the ECG graph paper equals:
    a. 0.20 seconds.
    b. 0.04 seconds.
    c. 1 second.
    d. 3 seconds.

12. Using the "3 to 5 rule," a sinus rhythm with four large boxes between each R-to-R interval would be:
    a. sinus tachycardia.
    b. sinus bradycardia.
    c. sinus arrest.
    d. normal sinus rhythm.

13. A normal sinus rhythm suddenly changes to an atrial tachycardia. This is called:
    a. abrupt transition.
    b. paroxysmal.
    c. autonomic tachycardia.
    d. chronotropic tachycardia.

14. The ventricles are not being completely filled with blood from the atria when:
    a. the QRS complex is absent.
    b. the R-to-R interval is irregular.
    c. the T wave is absent.
    d. the P wave is absent.

15. Junctional complexes can be identified by:
    a. inverted P waves.
    b. hidden P waves.
    c. P waves following the QRS.
    d. all of the above.

Practice Self-Test Answers

1.	b	6.	b	11.	a
2.	a	7.	a	12.	d
3.	c	8.	b	13.	b
4.	c	9.	e	14.	d
5.	d	10.	b	15.	d

CONTINUING EDUCATION CREDIT QUESTIONS

You must pass with at least 70% to earn 4 hours continuing education credit. Fill in the enclosed answer sheet and mail with your payment.

This program has been approved for 4.0 hours of nationally recognized continuing education credit for nurses (CEP#112446) and EMS providers (EMSA#33-0011) through Center for Healthcare Education, Inc. Successful participants will receive a certificate documenting continuing education hours within two weeks of receipt of application.

1. The term that describes PVCs with more than one configuration within the same ECG is:
   a. multifocal.
   b. unifocal.
   c. bigeminy.
   d. trigeminy.

2. Ventricular tachycardia is considered:
   a. normal in athletes and children.
   b. to be well tolerated.
   c. a lethal dysrhythmia.
   d. always benign.

3. Ideally, the initial treatment for VF is:
   a. epinephrine.
   b. atropine.
   c. defibrillation.
   d. synchronized cardioversion.

4. Ventricular dysrhythmias have what in common?
   a. Retrograde P-waves
   b. Inverted P-waves
   c. Wide QRS complexes
   d. Normal P-R intervals

5. Which AV block has a variable P-R interval?
   a. First-degree
   b. Second-degree type I
   c. Second-degree type II
   d. Fourth-degree

6. AV blocks typically have:
   a. a paroxysmal onset.
   b. rapid ventricular rates.
   c. slow ventricular rates.
   d. no P waves.

7. The inherent rate of the SA node is:
   a. 20 to 40 per minute.
   b. 40 to 60 per minute.
   c. 60 to 100 per minute.
   d. 100 to 140 per minute.

8. Blood flow returning from the body via the venous system first enters the heart through the:
   a. right atrium.
   b. right ventricle.
   c. left atrium.
   d. left ventricle.

9. The most common treatment for sinus tachycardia is:
   a. atropine.
   b. epinephrine.
   c. carotid massage.
   d. treatment for the underlying cause.

10. Which rhythm will most likely require emergency cardiac pacing?
    a. Third-degree AV block at a rate of 38 per minute
    b. Sinus tachycardia at a rate of 140 per minute
    c. Regular sinus rhythm at a rate of 68 per minute with frequent multifocal PVCs
    d. Atrial flutter at a rate of 58 per minute

11. Which of the following is *not* part of the five-step rhythm analysis?
    a. Count the rate
    b. Assess the rhythm
    c. Palpate the pulse
    d. Determine the P-to-QRS relationship

12. An upright deflection is seen on the ECG paper when the electrical impulse is traveling toward the:
    a. positive lead.
    b. negative lead.
    c. ground lead.
    d. isoelectric lead.

13. The "3 to 5 rule" indicates that the rhythm is most likely a/an:
    a. ventricular rhythm.
    b. atrial rhythm.
    c. regular sinus rhythm.
    d. junctional rhythm.

14. Heart rate is determined by evaluating the:
    a. P-to-QRS relationship.
    b. P-R interval.
    c. S-T segment.
    d. R-to-R interval.

15. A PAC (premature atrial complex) is an example of a/an:
    a. ectopic beat.
    b. escape beat.
    c. regular sinus beat.
    d. skipped beat.

True or False

16. The hallmark of atrial fibrillation is its chaotic wavy baseline and irregular R-to-R intervals.

17. The most effective treatment for third-degree AV block is usually a pacemaker.

18. First-degree block indicates a delay in conduction through the AV node.

19. Ectopic rhythms stem from an irritable focus.

20. Fibrillatory waves may be seen in both atrial and ventricular dysrhythmias.

21. If a patient has a pulse, it will be felt during the QRS complex.

22. The ECG provides information about the mechanical activity of the heart.

23. Sinus arrhythmia may be related to breathing.

24. A loose lead can mimic ventricular fibrillation or asystole.

25. In atrial fibrillation, the R-to-R intervals are usually irregular.

26. A patient can have a rhythm on the ECG and no pulse.

27. A regular sinus rhythm means that the patient is in no danger of having a myocardial infarction.

28. AV blocks always require a pacemaker.

29. The term *atrial kick* indicates that the atria are contracting and actively moving blood into the ventricles.

30. Another term for AV block Mobitz type I is *Wenckebach*.

For questions regarding continuing education credit please contact:

Continuing Education Division
Center for Healthcare Education, Inc.
3747 Arlington Ave.
Riverside, CA 92506
1-888-834-8700
www.healthcareeducation.org